# Summary

*Update: On June 20, 2012, the House of Representatives passed, by voice vote and under suspension of the rules, S. 3187 (EAH), the Food and Drug Administration Safety and Innovation Act, as amended. This bill would reauthorize the FDA prescription drug and medical device user fee programs (which would otherwise expire on September 30, 2012), create new user fee programs for generic and biosimilar drug approvals, and make other revisions to other FDA drug and device approval processes. It reflects bicameral compromise on earlier versions of the bill (S. 3187 [ES], which passed the Senate on May 24, 2012, and H.R. 5651 [EH], which passed the House on May 30, 2012). The following CRS reports provide overview information on FDA's processes for approval and regulation of drugs:*

- CRS Report R41983, *How FDA Approves Drugs and Regulates Their Safety and Effectiveness*, by Susan Thaul.

- CRS Report RL33986, *FDA's Authority to Ensure That Drugs Prescribed to Children Are Safe and Effective*, by Susan Thaul.

- CRS Report R42130, *FDA Regulation of Medical Devices*, by Judith A. Johnson.

- CRS Report R42508, *The FDA Medical Device User Fee Program*, by Judith A. Johnson.

*(Note: The rest of this report has not been updated since December 28, 2011.)*

Prior to and since the passage of the Medical Device Amendments of 1976, Congress has debated how best to ensure that consumers have access, as quickly as possible, to new and improved medical devices and, at the same time, prevent devices that are not safe and effective from entering or remaining on the market. Medical devices regulation is complex, in part, because of the wide variety of items that are categorized as medical devices; examples range from a simple tongue depressor to a life-sustaining heart valve. The regulation of medical devices can affect their cost, quality, and availability in the health care system.

In order to be legally marketed in the United States, many medical devices must be reviewed by the Food and Drug Administration (FDA), the agency responsible for protecting the public health by overseeing medical products, including devices. FDA's Center for Devices and Radiological Health (CDRH) is primarily responsible for medical device review. CDRH activities are funded through a combination of public money (i.e., direct FDA appropriations from Congress) and private money (i.e., user fees collected from device manufacturers) which together comprise FDA's total. User fees account for 33% of FDA's total FY2011 program level and 15% of CDRH's program level, which is $378 million in FY2011 including $56 million in user fees. FDA's authority to collect user fees, originally authorized in 2002 (P.L. 107-250), has been reauthorized in five-year increments. It will expire on October 1, 2012, under the terms of the Medical Device User Fee Act of 2007 (MDUFA), Title II of the FDA Amendments Act of 2007 (FDAAA, P.L. 110-85).

FDA requires all medical product manufacturers to register their facilities, list their devices with FDA, and follow general controls requirements. FDA classifies devices according to the risk they pose to consumers. Premarket review is required for moderate- and high-risk devices. There are two paths that manufacturers can use to bring such devices to market. One path consists of conducting clinical studies, submitting a *premarket approval* (PMA) application and requires evidence providing reasonable assurance that the device is safe and effective. The other path involves submitting a *510(k) notification* demonstrating that the device is *substantially equivalent* to a device already on the market (a *predicate device*) that does not require a PMA. The 510(k) process results in FDA *clearance* and tends to be much less expensive and less time-consuming than seeking FDA approval via PMA. Substantial equivalence is determined by comparing the performance characteristics of a new device with those of a predicate device; clinical data demonstrating safety and effectiveness are usually not required. Once approved or cleared for marketing, manufacturers must comply with regulations on manufacturing, labeling, surveillance, device tracking, and adverse event reporting.

Problems related to medical devices can have serious consequences for consumers. Defects in medical devices, such as artificial hips and pacemakers, have caused severe patient injuries and deaths. In 2006, FDA reported 116,086 device-related injuries, 96,485 malfunctions, and 2,830 deaths; an analysis by the National Research Center for Women & Families claims there were 4,556 device-related deaths in 2009. Reports published in 2009 through 2011—by the Government Accountability Office (GAO), the Department of Health and Human Services Office of the Inspector General and the Institute of Medicine—have voiced concerns about FDA's device review process. In 2009 and 2011 GAO included FDA's oversight of medical products on the GAO list of high-risk areas. FDA has conducted internal reviews as well and is implementing changes.

# Contents

Introduction............................................................................................................................... 1

The Medical Device Review Process: Premarket Requirements.................................................... 3

    Device Classification.......................................................................................................... 4

    Medical Device Marketing Applications.............................................................................. 7

        510(k) Notification..................................................................................................... 8

        Premarket Approval (PMA) ...................................................................................... 11

The Medical Device Review Process: Post-Market Requirements .............................................. 13

    Labeling.......................................................................................................................... 13

    Manufacturing ................................................................................................................ 14

    Postmarketing Surveillance ............................................................................................ 15

        Postmarket Surveillance........................................................................................... 15

        Adverse Event Reporting ......................................................................................... 15

        Medical Device Tracking .......................................................................................... 16

        The Sentinel Initiative .............................................................................................. 17

        Unique Device Identification .................................................................................... 18

    Compliance and Enforcement ......................................................................................... 19

        Inspection ................................................................................................................ 19

        Warning Letter.......................................................................................................... 20

        Product Recall .......................................................................................................... 20

# Tables

Table 1. Medical Device Classification ....................................................................................... 5

Table 2. CDRH, FDA Foreign and Domestic Inspections, FY2004–FY2010 ............................. 19

Table 3. CDRH Warning Letters Issued, FY2000–FY2010 ....................................................... 20

Table 4. CDRH Class I, II, and III Product Recalls, FY2004–FY2010 ...................................... 21

# Appendixes

Appendix A. History of Laws Governing Medical Device Regulation ......................................... 22

Appendix B. Acronyms Used in this Report............................................................................... 28

# Contacts

Author Contact Information........................................................................................................ 29

# Introduction

Update: On June 20, 2012, the House of Representatives passed, by voice vote and under suspension of the rules, S. 3187 (EAH), the Food and Drug Administration Safety and Innovation Act, as amended. This bill would reauthorize the FDA prescription drug and medical device user fee programs (which would otherwise expire on September 30, 2012), create new user fee programs for generic and biosimilar drug approvals, and make other revisions to other FDA drug and device approval processes. It reflects bicameral compromise on earlier versions of the bill (S. 3187 [ES], which passed the Senate on May 24, 2012, and HR 5651 [EH], which passed the House on May 30, 2012). The following CRS reports provide overview information on FDA's processes for approval and regulation of drugs:

- CRS Report R41983, *How FDA Approves Drugs and Regulates Their Safety and Effectiveness*, by Susan Thaul.

- CRS Report RL33986, *FDA's Authority to Ensure That Drugs Prescribed to Children Are Safe and Effective*, by Susan Thaul.

- CRS Report R42130, *FDA Regulation of Medical Devices*, by Judith A. Johnson.

- CRS Report R42508, *The FDA Medical Device User Fee Program*, by Judith A. Johnson.

(Note: The rest of this report has not been updated since December 28, 2011.)

Medical device regulation is complex, in part because of the wide variety of items that are categorized as medical devices. They may be simple tools used during medical examinations, such as tongue depressors and thermometers, or high-tech life-saving implants like heart valves and coronary stents. The medical device market has been characterized as including eight industry sectors: surgical and medical instrument manufacturing, surgical appliance and supplies, in vitro diagnostic products (IVDs, or laboratory tests), electromedical and electrotherapeutic apparatus, irradiation apparatus, dental equipment and supplies, ophthalmic goods, and dental laboratories.[1]

The federal agency primarily responsible for regulating medical devices is the Food and Drug Administration (FDA)—an agency within the Department of Health and Human Services (HHS). A manufacturer must receive FDA permission before its device can be legally marketed in the United States. FDA's Center for Devices and Radiological Health (CDRH) is primarily responsible for medical device review. Another center, the Center for Biologics Evaluation and Research (CBER), regulates devices associated with blood collection and processing procedures, cellular products and tissues.[2]

CDRH activities are funded through a combination of public money (i.e., direct FDA appropriations from Congress) and private money (i.e., user fees collected from device manufacturers) which together comprise FDA's total.[3] User fees may be used only to support product review activities, not other CDRH activities. User fees account for 33% of FDA's total FY2011 program level and 15% of CDRH's program level, which is $378 million in FY2011 including $56 million in user fees.[4] Congress has reauthorized in five-year increments FDA

---

[1] The Lewin Group, for AdvaMed, *State Economic Impact of the Medical Technology Industry*, June 7, 2010, p. 19.

[2] Jurisdiction of the centers' medical device review is governed by the FDA Intercenter Agreement between CBER and CDRH (October 31, 1991). FDA, *Devices Regulated by the Center for Biologics Evaluation and Research*, http://www.fda.gov/BiologicsBloodVaccines/DevelopmentApprovalProcess/510kProcess/ucm133429.htm.

[3] For more information on FDA's budget, see CRS Report R41737, *Public Health Service (PHS) Agencies Overview and Funding, FY2010-FY2012*, coordinated by C. Stephen Redhead and Pamela W. Smith; and, CRS Report RL34334, *The Food and Drug Administration Budget and Statutory History, FY1980-FY2007*, coordinated by Judith A. Johnson.

[4] FDA also funds some device and radiological health activities with fees collected under the Mammography Quality (continued...)

collection of medical device user fees; authority will expire on October 1, 2012 under the terms of the Medical Device User Fee Act of 2007 (MDUFA), Title II of the FDA Amendments Act of 2007 (FDAAA, P.L. 110-85).

Congress has historically been interested in balancing the goals of allowing consumers to have access, as quickly as possible, to new and improved medical devices with preventing devices that are not safe and effective from entering or remaining on the market. The goals of device availability and device safety may exert opposite pulls, with implications for consumers, the health care system, and the economy.

Investment in medical device development reportedly reached a high of $3.690 billion in 2007. Investment has slowed somewhat to $2.380 billion in 2010, and $1.510 billion in the first two quarters of 2011.[5] According to one report, the medical technology industry is a "vibrant and growing contributor to the U.S. economy, generating US$197 billion in revenue and employing over a half million workers in 2009 alone."[6] "Medical technology industry" includes "medical device, diagnostic, drug delivery and analytic/life science tool companies but excludes distributors and service providers" such as contract research or contract manufacturing organizations.[7] Another analysis found that "32 of the 46 medical technology companies with more than $1 billion in annual revenue are based in the United States."[8] Although the largest companies dominate the market for devices in terms of sales, it is often the small device companies that make a significant contribution to early innovation. Small companies may partner with larger companies to bring products to market if they lack access to the capital and resources to conduct clinical trials and navigate regulatory and reimbursement hurdles.

Manufacturers make decisions about pursuing new devices based in part on the cost of their development. Additional regulatory requirements may escalate these costs, while other incentives, such as tax breaks or market exclusivity extensions, may diminish them. If the device development cost is too high, the eventual result may be that consumers are denied access because new products are not developed or brought to market. Access problems have led to proposals for, and the enactment of, incentives to develop medical devices for rare diseases and pediatric populations. However, if the regulation and oversight of device development are not stringent enough, unsafe or ineffective products may reach the market and cause harm to consumers.

Problems related to medical devices can have serious consequences for consumers. Defects in medical devices, such as artificial hips, pacemakers, defibrillators, and stents, have caused severe patient injuries and deaths.[9] In 2006, FDA reported 116,086 device-related injuries, 96,485

---

(...continued)

Standards Act (MQSA, P.L. 102-539), and device user fees fund some non–device-specific activities at FDA.

[5] PriceWaterhouseCoopers / National Venture Capital Association, "Medical Devices and Equipment," *Money Tree Report*, data provided by Thomson Reuters, at http://www.pwcmoneytree.com.

[6] Ernst and Young. 2010. *Pulse of the industry  Medical technology report*, p. 15.

[7] Ibid., p. 87.

[8] PwC (PricewaterhouseCoopers), *Medical Technology Innovation Scorecard  The race for global leadership*, January 2011, p. 8, http://www.pwc.com/us/en/health-industries/health-research-institute/innovation-scorecard.

[9] For example, see Barry Meier and Janet Roberts, "Hip implant complaints surge, even as the dangers are studied," *The New York Times*, August 22, 2011, pp. A1, A16; Information on recalls is available by searching the database at FDA, *Medical & Radiation Emitting Device Recalls*, http://www.accessdata.fda.gov/scripts/cdrh/cfdocs/cfRES/res.cfm.

malfunctions, and 2,830 deaths; a more recent independent analysis claims there were 4,556 device-related deaths in 2009.[10] Consequences such as these have raised questions as to whether adequate enforcement tools, resources, and processes are in place to ensure that marketed devices are safe. Reports by the Government Accountability Office (GAO), the Department of Health and Human Services Office of the Inspector General, and the Institute of Medicine (IOM) have voiced concerns about FDA's device review process.[11] In 2009 and in 2011 GAO included FDA's oversight of medical products on the GAO list of high-risk areas.[12]

This report provides a description of FDA's medical device review process divided into two parts: premarket requirements and postmarket requirements. **Appendix A** provides a brief history of laws governing medical device regulation and **Appendix B** provides a table of acronyms used in the report.

## The Medical Device Review Process: Premarket Requirements

FDA requires all medical product manufacturers to register their facilities, list their devices with the agency, and follow general controls requirements.[13] FDA classifies devices according to the risk they pose to consumers. Many medical devices, such as plastic bandages and ice bags, present only minimal risk and can be legally marketed upon registration alone. These low-risk devices are deemed *exempt* from premarket review and manufacturers need not submit an application to FDA prior to marketing.[14] In contrast, most moderate- and high-risk devices must obtain the agency's permission prior to marketing. FDA grants this permission when a manufacturer meets regulatory premarket requirements and agrees to any necessary postmarket requirements which vary according to the risk that a device presents.[15]

---

**PMA vs. 510(k)**

There is a fundamental difference between the PMA and 510(k) pathways. In a PMA review, FDA determines if the device is reasonably safe and effective for its intended use. In a 510(k) review, FDA determines if the device is substantially equivalent to another device whose safety and effectiveness may never have been assessed.

---

[10] FDA, CDRH Reports, OCD FY2006: FDA Goal 3-Improving Product Quality, Safety, and Availability Through Better Manufacturing and Product Oversight, at http://www.fda.gov/AboutFDA/CentersOffices/CDRH/CDRHReports/ucm129324.htm; and Statement of Diana Zuckerman, PhD, President of the National Research Center for Women & Families at the House of Representatives Briefing on Medical Devices, May 17, 2011, at http://www.center4research.org/2011/05/statement-of-diana-zuckerman-phd-president-of-the-national-research-center-for-women-families-at-a-house-of-representatives-briefing-on-medical-devices/.

[11] U.S. Government Accountability Office, *Medical Devices FDA should take steps to ensure that high-risk device types are approved through the most stringent premarket review process*, GAO-09-190, January 2009; Daniel R. Levinson, *Adverse Event Reporting for Medical Devices*, Department of Health and Human Services, Office of Inspector General, Washington, DC, October 2009; and, IOM (Institute of Medicine), *Medical Devices and the Public's Health The FDA 510(k) Clearance Process at 35 Years*, Washington, DC, July 2011.

[12] GAO regularly reports on government operations that it identifies as high risk due to their greater vulnerability to fraud, waste, abuse, mismanagement or the need for transformation to address economy, efficiency or effectiveness challenges. See GAO, *High-Risk Series An Update*, GAO-09-271, January 2009; and GAO, *High-Risk Series An Update*, GAO-11-278, February 2011.

[13] (21 CFR 862-892).

[14] The term *manufacturer* is used throughout this report for simplicity, but regulations also apply to any person, organization, or sponsor that submits an application to FDA to market a device.

[15] *In vitro* diagnostic products (IVDs, or laboratory tests) have their own unique premarket requirements and are not (continued...)

---

There are two paths that manufacturers can use to bring their moderate- and high-risk devices to market with FDA's permission. One path consists of conducting clinical studies, submitting a *premarket approval* (PMA) application and requires evidence providing reasonable assurance that the device is safe and effective.[16] The PMA process is generally used for novel and high-risk devices and is typically lengthy and expensive. It results in a type of FDA permission called *approval.*

The other path involves submitting a *510(k) notification* demonstrating that the device is *substantially equivalent* to a device already on the market (a *predicate device*) that does not require a PMA.[17] The 510(k) process is unique to medical devices and results in FDA *clearance.* Substantial equivalence is determined by comparing the performance characteristics of a new device with those of a predicate device. To be considered substantially equivalent, the new device must have the same intended use and technological characteristics as the predicate; clinical data demonstrating safety and effectiveness are usually not required. The manufacturer selects the predicate device to compare with its new device. However, FDA has the ultimate discretion in determining whether a comparison is appropriate.

According to a 2009 GAO report, of the more than 50,000 devices that were listed by manufacturers with FDA from FY2003 through FY2007, about 67% were exempt from premarket review; the remainder entered the market via the 510(k) process (31%), the PMA process (1%) or via other means.[18]

## Device Classification

Under the terms of the Medical Device Amendments of 1976 (MDA, P.L. 94-295), FDA classified all medical devices that were on the market at the time of enactment—the *preamendment* devices—into one of three classes. Congress provided definitions for the three classes—Class I, Class II, Class III—based on the risk (low-, moderate-, and high-risk respectively) to patients posed by the devices.[19] Examples of each class are listed in **Table 1**. Device classification determines the type of regulatory requirements that a manufacturer must follow. Regulatory requirements for each class are described below in more detail. *General controls*, the minimum regulations that apply to all FDA regulated medical devices, include five elements:[20]

---

(...continued)

discussed further in this report.

[16] This is somewhat similar to the process FDA uses to approve a new prescription drug. For more information, see CRS Report R41983, *How FDA Approves Drugs and Regulates Their Safety and Effectiveness,* by Susan Thaul.

[17] To be a predicate, a device must have either been on the market before 1976 when the Medical Device Amendments (MDA) took effect, or it could have been cleared for marketing after 1976, but must have the same intended use as a device classified in the Code of Federal Regulations (CFR).

[18] U.S. Government Accountability Office, *Medical Devices FDA should take steps to ensure that high-risk device types are approved through the most stringent premarket review process,* GAO-09-190, January 2009, p. 9.

[19] FFDCA §513(a)(1); see also 21 CFR §860.3(c). As of 2009, the agency has classified over 1,700 distinct types of devices. The device types are organized in the Code of Federal Regulations (CFR) in 16 *classification panels,* such as "cardiovascular devices" or "ear, nose, and throat devices." FDA, *Device Classification,* June 18, 2009, http://www.fda.gov/MedicalDevices/DeviceRegulationandGuidance/Overview/ClassifyYourDevice/default.htm.

[20] See FDA, *General and Special Controls,* April 30, 2009, http://www.fda.gov/MedicalDevices/DeviceRegulationandGuidance/Overview/GeneralandSpecialControls/default.htm.

---

- *establishment registration*—such as manufacturers, distributors, repackagers and relabelers, and foreign firms;[21]

- *device listing*—listing with FDA of all devices to be marketed;

- good manufacturing practices (GMP)—manufacturing of devices in accordance with the Quality Systems Regulation (QSR);[22]

- *labeling*—labeling of devices or in vitro diagnostic products;[23] and

- *premarket notification*—submission to FDA of a premarket notification 510(k).

### Table 1. Medical Device Classification

| Device Classification | Examples | Safety / Effectiveness Controls | Required Submission |
| --- | --- | --- | --- |
| Class I | elastic bandages, examination gloves, and hand-held surgical instruments | General Controls | -*Registration only* unless 510(k) specifically required |
| Class II | powered wheelchairs, infusion pumps, and surgical drapes | General Controls & Special Controls | -*510(k) clearance* unless exempt<br>-*IDE possible* |
| Class III | heart valves, silicone gel-filled breast implants, and implanted cerebella stimulators | General Controls & Premarket Approval | -*PMA approval*<br>-*IDE probable* |
| | metal-on-metal hip joint, certain dental implants | General Controls | -*510(k) clearance* |

**Source**: FDA, Overview of Medical Device Regulation, General and Special Controls, at http://www.fda.gov/MedicalDevices/DeviceRegulationandGuidance/Overview/GeneralandSpecialControls/default.htm.

**Note:** IDE means investigational device exemption.

**Class I** devices are those under current law for which general controls "are sufficient to provide reasonable assurance of the safety and effectiveness of the device."[24] Many Class I devices are *exempt* from the premarket notification and/or the QSR requirements, though they still have to comply with the other general controls. A device is exempt if FDA determines that it presents a low risk of illness or injury to patients.[25]

**Class II** devices are those under current law "which cannot be classified as class I because the general controls by themselves are insufficient to provide reasonable assurance of safety and effectiveness of the device."[26] Class II includes devices that pose a moderate risk to patients, and may include new devices for which information or *special controls* are available to reduce or mitigate risk. Special controls may include special labeling requirements, mandatory performance standards, and postmarket surveillance. Currently "15% of all device types classified in Class II

---

[21] 21 CFR 807.20

[22] 21 CFR 820

[23] 21 CFR 801 or 809.10.

[24] FFDCA §513(a)(1)(A).

[25] See 21 CFR 862 to 892.

[26] FFDCA §513(a)(1)(B).

are subject to special controls."[27] Although most Class II devices require premarket notification via the 510(k) process, a few are exempt by regulation.[28]

**Class III** devices are those under current law which "cannot be classified as a class I device because insufficient information exists to determine that the application of general controls are sufficient to provide reasonable assurance of the safety and effectiveness of the device," and "cannot be classified as a class II device because insufficient information exists to determine that the special controls ... would provide reasonable assurance of [their] safety and effectiveness," and are "purported or represented to be for a use in supporting or sustaining human life or for a use which is of substantial importance in preventing impairment of human health," or present "a potential unreasonable risk of illness or injury, [are] to be subject ... to premarket approval to provide reasonable assurance of [their] safety and effectiveness."[29]

In other words, general and/or special controls are not sufficient to assure safe and effective use of a Class III device. Class III includes devices which are life-supporting or life-sustaining, and devices which present a high or potentially unreasonable risk of illness or injury to a patient. New devices that are not classified as Class I or II by another means, are automatically designated as Class III unless the manufacturer files a request or petition for reclassification.[30]

Although most Class III devices require *premarket approval* (PMA), some Class III devices may be cleared via the 510(k) process. In fact, during the first 10 years following enactment of MDA, over 80% of postamendment Class III devices entered the market on the basis of 510(k) submissions showing substantial equivalence to preamendment devices.[31] According to FDA, these are "postamendment (i.e., introduced to the U.S. market after May 28, 1976) Class III devices which are substantially equivalent to preamendment (i.e., introduced to the U.S. market before May 28, 1976) Class III devices and for which the regulation calling for the premarket approval application has not been published in 21 CFR."[32] FDA explains the situation as follows:

> When FDA's medical device regulation program began in the late 1970s, FDA regulated over 100 Class III device types through the 510(k) program. The intent was that FDA's regulation would be temporary and that over time, FDA would decide to reclassify those device types (or regulations) into Class I or II, or to sustain the classification in Class III and call for PMA applications. The process of reclassification is described in FDA's regulations in Section 515 of the Federal Food, Drug and Cosmetic Act. Over the years, FDA has made progress in this original list; however, as of 2009, 26 medical device regulations remained in this transitional state awaiting final classification.[33]

---

[27] IOM, *Medical Devices and the Public's Health The FDA 510(k) Clearance Process at 35 Years*, Washington, DC, July 2011, p. 40.

[28] FDA, Overview of Medical Device Regulation, Medical Device Classification, Class I/II Exemptions, at http://www.fda.gov/MedicalDevices/DeviceRegulationandGuidance/Overview/ClassifyYourDevice/ucm051549.htm.

[29] FFDCA §513(a)(1)(C).

[30] FFDCA §513(f)(2).

[31] IOM, *Medical Devices and the Public's Health The FDA 510(k) Clearance Process at 35 Years*, Washington, DC, July 2011, p. 81.

[32] FDA, Overview of Medical Device Regulation, General and Special Controls, at http://www.fda.gov/MedicalDevices/DeviceRegulationandGuidance/Overview/GeneralandSpecialControls/default.htm.

[33] FDA, CDRH Transparency, 515 Program Initiative, at http://www.fda.gov/AboutFDA/CentersOffices/CDRH/CDRHTransparency/ucm240310.htm.

---

At the time that the MDA of 1976 was drafted, "relatively few medical devices were permanently implanted or intended to sustain life. The 510(k) process was specifically intended for devices with less need for scientific scrutiny, such as surgical gloves and hearing aids."[34] Over time, FDA's 510(k) review process was "challenged as new devices changed more dramatically and became more complex."[35]

Examples of Class III devices that are still regulated via the 510(k) program include the metal-on-metal hip joint, certain dental implants, automated external defibrillator, electroconvulsive therapy device, pedicle screw spinal system, intra-aortic balloon and control system, and several device types related to pacemakers.[36] In late 2009, FDA implemented the 515 Program Initiative "to facilitate the final adjudication of these remaining Class III device types."[37]

## Medical Device Marketing Applications

As stated above, in general, before a non-exempt medical device may be legally marketed, a manufacturer must submit to FDA either: a PMA application, and the agency *approves* the device; or, a 510(k) notification, and the agency *clears* the device. FDA makes its determination—either approval or clearance—based on information the manufacturer submits. The information that is required—in other words, the type of marketing application the manufacturer must make (if any)—is determined based on the *risk* that the device poses, if used according to the manufacturer's instructions. FDA typically evaluates more than 4,000 510(k) notifications and about 40 original PMA applications each year.[38]

The Food and Drug Administration Modernization Act of 1997 (FDAMA; P.L. 105-115) gave FDA the authority to establish procedures for meeting with manufacturers prior to preparing a submission.[39] The procedures aim to speed the review process by giving FDA and a manufacturer the opportunity to address questions and concerns about the device and/or the planned studies that will be used to support the marketing application before the studies are initiated and the application is submitted. Requests for these meetings have doubled over the past five years according to testimony by CDRH Director Jeffrey Shuren at a November 2011 Senate hearing.[40]

---

[34] Diana M. Zuckerman, Paul Brown, and Steven Nissen, "Medical device recalls and the FDA approval process," *Archives of Internal Medicine*, Online publication 2011, p. E2.

[35] Ibid., p. E2.

[36] FDA, CDRH Transparency, 515 Program Status, at http://www.fda.gov/AboutFDA/CentersOffices/CDRH/ CDRHTransparency/ucm240318.htm.

[37] FDA, CDRH Transparency, 515 Program Initiative, at http://www.fda.gov/AboutFDA/CentersOffices/CDRH/ CDRHTransparency/ucm240310.htm.

[38] U.S. Congress, Senate Special Committee on Aging, *A Delicate Balance FDA and the Reform of the Medical Device Approval Process*, Testimony of William Maisel, Deputy Center Director for Science, FDA/CDRH, 112th Cong., 1st sess., April 13, 2011.

[39] For guidance on the procedures established, see *Early Collaboration Meetings Under the FDA Modernization Act*; Final Guidance for Industry and CDRH Staff, February 28, 2001, at http://www.fda.gov/MedicalDevices/ DeviceRegulationandGuidance/GuidanceDocuments/ucm073604.htm.

[40] U.S. Congress, Senate Committee on Health, Education, Labor, and Pensions, *Medical Devices Protecting Patients and Promoting Innovation*, 112th Cong., 1st sess., November 15, 2011.

---

Generally speaking, under the Federal Food, Drug and Cosmetic Act (FFDCA), manufacturers

- are prohibited from selling an adulterated product;[41]
- are prohibited from misbranding a product;[42]
- must register their facility with FDA and list all of the medical devices that they produce or process (and a fee is now required under the terms of FDAAA);
- must file the appropriate premarket submission with the agency at least 90 days before introducing a *non-exempt* device onto the market; and
- must report to FDA any incident that they are aware of that suggests that their device may have caused or contributed to a death or serious injury.

Under the terms of MDUFA (Title II of FDAAA), manufacturers must pay a fee for most types of submissions. In 2010, FDA charged $217,787 in user fees to review a PMA ($54,447 for smaller companies) and $4,007 to review a 510(k) submission ($2,004 for small companies).[43] GAO found that in 2005, the average cost for FDA to review a PMA was $870,000 and the average cost to review a 510(k) submission was $18,200.[44] According to CDRH Director Jeffrey Shuren, user fees collected under MDUFA "fund only about 20% of the device review program;" in contrast, users fees collected under the Prescription Drug User Fee Act (PDUFA) "account for about two-thirds of the drug review program's budget."[45]

## 510(k) Notification

In general, a 510(k) submission is required for a moderate-risk medical device that is not non-exempt from premarket review. A 510(k) could also be used for currently marketed devices for which the manufacturer seeks a new indication (e.g., a new population, such as pediatric use, or a new disease or condition), or for which the manufacturer has changed the design or technical characteristics such that the change may affect the performance characteristics of the device.

Between 1996 and 2009, more than 80% of the devices cleared by FDA using 510(k) notification were Class II devices, about 10% were Class I and less than 5% were Class III.[46] A 2009 GAO report found that 25% of the 10,670 Class II devices cleared by FDA in FY2003 through FY2007

---

[41] A device is adulterated if it includes any filthy, putrid, or decomposed substance, or if it is prepared, packed, or held under unsanitary conditions. The FFDCA further states that a device is adulterated if its container contains any poisonous or deleterious substance, or if its strength, purity or quality varies significantly from what the manufacturer claims. For higher class devices, a device can be considered adulterated if it fails to meet performance requirements outlined in its approval, or if it is in violation of other Good Manufacturing Practice requirements.

[42] A device is misbranded when all or part of the labeling (i.e., the FDA-approved printed material providing information about the device) is false, misleading, or missing.

[43] FDA, "Medical Device User Fee Rates for Fiscal Year 2010," 74 *Federal Register* 38444-38449, August 3, 2009; http://edocket.access.gpo.gov/2009/E9-18456.htm.

[44] U.S. Government Accountability Office, *Medical Devices FDA should take steps to ensure that high-risk device types are approved through the most stringent premarket review process*, GAO-09-190, January 2009.

[45] U.S. Congress, Senate Committee on Health, Education, Labor, and Pensions, *Medical Devices Protecting Patients and Promoting Innovation*, Testimony of Jeffrey Shuren, Director CDRH, FDA, 112th Cong., 1st sess., November 15, 2011, http://help.senate.gov/imo/media/doc/Shuren.pdf.

[46] IOM, *Public Health Effectiveness of the FDA 510(k) Clearance Process Measuring Postmarket Performance and Other Select Topics*, Workshop Report, Washington, DC, 2011, pp. 12 and 78.

---

were either implantable, life sustaining or presented significant risk to the health, safety, or welfare of the patient.[47] The agency cleared about 90% of 510(k) submissions reviewed during FY2003 through FY2007.[48]

As noted previously, the standard for clearance of a traditional 510(k) is substantial equivalence with a predicate device. A predicate device can be one of two things. It can be a previously cleared Class I or II device that does not require a PMA. It can also be preamendment Class III for which the agency has not issued regulations requiring a PMA. (PMAs, which are more rigorous submissions than 510(k)s, are discussed in the "Premarket Approval (PMA)" section.)

A manufacturer may choose one of three types of 510(k) submissions for premarket clearance: traditional, special, or abbreviated.[49] A study of 510(k) submissions between 1996 and 2009 found that about 80% were traditional, 16% were special, and 3% were abbreviated.[50] For novel devices without a predicate, there is another alternative called the de novo 510(k) process.

In a traditional 510(k), the manufacturer submits information about the

> **2011 IOM Report on 510(k) Substantial Equivalence**
>
> "In practice, the assessment of substantial equivalence generally does not require evidence of safety or effectiveness of a device. Unlike the premarket approval (PMA) process, by law the 510(k) process, with some exceptions [see SMDA 1990], focuses solely on the determination of a device's substantial equivalence to a predicate device. According to the FDA and the Supreme Court, when the FDA finds a device substantially equivalent to a predicate device, it has done no more than find that the new device is as safe and effective as the predicate. It is important to note that devices on the market before the enactment of the 1976 Medical Device Amendments (MDA)—the origin of all predicate devices for the 510(k) process—have never been systematically assessed to determine their safety and effectiveness. Because the preamendment device to which equivalence was established was not itself reviewed for safety or effectiveness, the committee found that clearance of a 510(k) submission was not a determination that the cleared device was safe or effective." See p. 154.

performance of the device under specific conditions of use. It also contains information about the design of the device, characteristics of device components, representations of packaging and labeling, a description and summary of the non-clinical and clinical studies that were done to support the device performance characteristics, a description of means by which users can assess the quality of the device, and information about any computer software or additional or special equipment needed. Several administrative forms are also required.[51]

Most of the studies supporting a 510(k) submission are not clinical studies. Substantial equivalence, in many cases, means only that the device performs in a similar fashion to the predicate under a similar set of circumstances. As a result, many devices never have to demonstrate safety and effectiveness through clinical studies.

---

[47] U.S. Government Accountability Office, *Medical Devices FDA should take steps to ensure that high-risk device types are approved through the most stringent premarket review process*, GAO-09-190, January 2009, p. 18.

[48] Ibid., p. 27.

[49] FDA, Medical Devices, 510(k) Submission Methods, at http://www.fda.gov/MedicalDevices/DeviceRegulationandGuidance/HowtoMarketYourDevice/PremarketSubmissions/PremarketNotification510k/ucm134034.htm

[50] IOM, *Public Health Effectiveness of the FDA 510(k) Clearance Process Measuring Postmarket Performance and Other Select Topics*, Workshop Report, Washington, DC, 2011, pp. 12 and 79.

[51] FDA, *How to Prepare a Traditional 510(k)*, September 14, 2009; http://www.fda.gov/MedicalDevices/DeviceRegulationandGuidance/HowtoMarketYourDevice/PremarketSubmissions/PremarketNotification510k/ucm134572.htm#link_4.

In addition to not requiring clinical studies, three other characteristics of the 510(k) process make it much less rigorous than the PMA process: (1) premarket inspections of how devices were manufactured are generally not required by FDA; (2) postmarket studies are not required by FDA as a condition of clearance; and, (3) FDA has limited authority to rescind or withdraw clearance if a 510(k) device is found to be unsafe or ineffective.[52]

FDA may take any of the following actions on a 510(k) after conducting its review:

- find the device substantially equivalent to the predicate and issue a clearance letter;

- find the device not substantially equivalent (NSE) and issue an NSE letter prohibiting marketing;

- determine that the device is exempt from a 510(k) submission;

- request additional information (with the final clearance decision pending review of that information).[53]

A manufacturer generally has 30 days to provide any additional information, or FDA may issue a notice of withdrawal of the application.54 The manufacturer may, at any time, withdraw its 510(k). FDA has 90 days to review a traditional 510(k).[55]

Abbreviated and special 510(k)s were new approaches to premarket notification that came from FDAMA. These approaches were intended to streamline and expedite FDA's review for routine submissions meeting certain qualifications, thus leaving reviewer time for more complicated submissions.

An abbreviated 510(k) uses guidance documents developed by FDA to communicate regulatory and scientific expectations to industry. Guidance documents have been prepared for many different kinds of devices, and are available on FDA's website. All guidance documents are developed in accordance with Good Guidance Practices (GGP), and many with public participation or opportunities for public comment.[56] In addition to issuing guidance documents, FDA can either develop performance or consensus standards or 'recognize' those developed by outside parties.[57] In an abbreviated 510(k), the manufacturer describes what guidance document, special control, or performance standard was used, and how it was used to assess performance of their device. Other minimum required elements are the product description, representative labeling, and a summary of the performance characteristics. FDA typically reviews an abbreviated 510(k) in 60 days.

---

[52] Diana M. Zuckerman, Paul Brown, and Steven Nissen, "Medical device recalls and the FDA approval process," *Archives of Internal Medicine*, Online publication 2011, p. E4.

[53] 21 CFR 807.100(a).

[54] 21 CFR 807.87(l).

[55] The FDA time clock (i.e., review cycle) begins when FDA receives the 510(k) and ends with the date that FDA issues either a request for additional information or a decision. More than one cycle may occur before FDA issues its final decision.

[56] 21 CFR 10.115. FDA continually accepts public comment on any draft or final guidance document.

[57] 21 CFR 861.

A special 510(k) may be used for a modification to a device that has already been cleared; it typically uses the design control[58] requirement of the Quality System Regulation (QSR). The QSR describes the good manufacturing practice (GMP) requirements for medical devices.[59] The special 510(k) allows the manufacturer to declare conformance to design controls without providing the data. This type of submission references the original 510(k) number, and contains information about the design control requirements. FDA aims to review most special 510(k)s in 30 days.

Under the FFDCA, novel devices lacking a legally marketed predicate are automatically designated Class III. FDAMA amended FFDCA Section 513(f) to allow FDA to establish a new, expedited mechanism for reclassifying these devices based on risk, thus reducing the regulatory burden on manufacturers. The de novo 510(k), though requiring more data than a traditional 510(k), often requires less information than a premarket approval (PMA) application.

In a de novo 510(k) process, the manufacturer submits a traditional 510(k) for its device. However, because there is no predicate device or classification, the agency will return a decision of not substantially equivalent. Within 30 days, the manufacturer submits a petition requesting reclassification of its device into Class II or I, as appropriate. Within 60 days, FDA will render a decision classifying the device according to criteria in FFDCA Section 513(a)(1). With approval, FDA issues a regulation that classifies the device. If the device is Class II, a special controls guidance document is also developed that then allows subsequent manufacturers to submit either traditional or abbreviated 510(k)s.[60] On September 30, 2011, FDA released draft guidance designed to further streamline the de novo review process.[61]

## Premarket Approval (PMA)

A PMA is the most stringent type of device marketing application required by FDA for new and/or high-risk devices. PMA approval is based on a determination by FDA that the application contains sufficient valid scientific evidence to assure that the device is safe and effective for its intended use(s).[62] In contrast to a 510(k), PMAs generally require some clinical data prior to gaining approval.[63] All clinical evaluations of investigational devices (unless exempt) must have an investigational device exemption (IDE) before the study is initiated.[64] An IDE allows an

---

[58] Design controls are a series of predetermined checks, verifications, and specifications that are built into the manufacturing process to validate the quality of the product throughout the process. These can include defining the personnel responsible for implementing steps in the development and manufacturing process, defining specifications and standards for assessing the quality of the materials that go into making the product, designing specifications for accepting and rejecting different batches or lots of final product, and requirements for maintaining appropriate records.

[59] 21 CFR 820.30.

[60] FDA, *New Section 513(f)(2)—Evaluation of Automatic Class III Designation, Guidance for Industry and CDRH Staff*, February 19, 1998, http://www.fda.gov/MedicalDevices/DeviceRegulationandGuidance/GuidanceDocuments/ucm080195.htm.

[61] Food and Drug Administration, "FDA Seeks Comment on Streamlined Review of Lower Risk, New Technology, Devices," press release, September 30, 2011, http://www.fda.gov/NewsEvents/Newsroom/PressAnnouncements/ucm274008.htm.

[62] 21 CFR 814.

[63] PMAs can also use studies from the medical literature (a "paper PMA").

[64] See 21 CFR 812. Devices are exempt from IDE requirements when testing is noninvasive, does not require invasive sampling, does not introduce energy into a subject, and is not stand alone (i.e., is not used for diagnosis without confirmation by other methods or medically established procedures). See 21 CFR 812.2(c)(3).

---

unapproved device (most commonly an invasive or life-sustaining device) to be used in a clinical study to collect the data required to support a PMA submission.[65] The IDE permits a device to be shipped lawfully for investigation of the device without requiring that the manufacturer comply with other requirements of the FFDCA, such as registration and listing. In August and in November 2011 FDA released new draft guidance intended to ensure the quality of clinical trials and streamline the IDE process by clarifying the criteria for approving clinical trials.[66] All clinical studies must also receive prior approval by an institutional review board (IRB).[67]

A PMA must contain (among other things) the following information:

- summaries of non-clinical and clinical data supporting the intended use and performance characteristics;

- detailed information on the device design and device components;

- instructions for use;

- representations of packaging and labeling;

- a description of means by which users can assess the quality of the device;

- information about computer software or additional or special equipment;

- literature about the disease and the similar devices; and,

- information on the manufacturing process.

Approval is based not only on the strength of the scientific data, but also on inspection of the manufacturing facility to assure that the facility and the manufacturing process are in compliance with the quality systems regulations (QSR).[68] FDAMA made it easier for manufacturers to submit the required sections of a PMA in a serial fashion as data are available ("modular PMA").

When a PMA is first received, FDA has 45 days to make sure the application is administratively complete. If not, the application is returned. If the application is complete, it is formally filed by FDA. The agency then has 75 days to complete the initial review and determine whether an advisory committee meeting will be necessary.

Advisory committees can be convened to make recommendations on any scientific or policy matter before FDA.[69] They are comprised of scientific, medical, and statistical experts, and industry and consumer representatives. An advisory committee meeting allows interested persons

---

[65] FDA, *Device Advice  Investigational Device Exemption (IDE)*, July 9, 2009, http://www.fda.gov/MedicalDevices/DeviceRegulationandGuidance/HowtoMarketYourDevice/InvestigationalDeviceExemptionIDE/default.htm.

[66] FDA, "FDA seeks comment on proposed guidance for high-quality clinical studies," FDA, press release, August 15, 2011, http://www.fda.gov/NewsEvents/Newsroom/PressAnnouncements/ucm268000 htm; and, "FDA issues two draft guidance documents to facilitate investigational medical device studies in humans," press release, November 10, 2011, http://www.fda.gov/NewsEvents/Newsroom/PressAnnouncements/ucm279459.htm.

[67] An IRB is a group, generally comprised volunteers, that examines proposed and ongoing scientific research to ensure that human subjects are properly protected. For further information, see CRS Report RL32909, *Federal Protection for Human Research Subjects  An Analysis of the Common Rule and Its Interactions with FDA Regulations and the HIPAA Privacy Rule*, by Erin D. Williams.

[68] 21 CFR 820.

[69] For further information, see CRS Report RS22691, *FDA Advisory Committee Conflict of Interest*, by Erin D. Williams.

---

to present information and views at a public hearing.[70] FDA typically accepts advisory committee recommendations for an application (approvable, approvable with conditions, or non-approvable). However, there have been cases where FDA's decision has not been consistent with the committee's recommendation. CDRH will hold joint advisory committee meetings with other centers where necessary.

After FDA notifies the applicant that the PMA has been approved or denied, a notice may be published on the Internet announcing the data on which the decision is based and providing interested persons an opportunity to petition FDA within 30 days for reconsideration of the decision. Though FDA regulations allow 180 days to review the PMA and make a determination, total review time can be much longer.[71] MDUFA performance goals have been established to reduce the review time for PMAs.[72]

# The Medical Device Review Process: Post-Market Requirements

Once approved or cleared for marketing, manufacturers of medical devices must comply with various regulations on labeling and advertising, manufacturing, postmarketing surveillance, device tracking, and adverse event reporting. This section describes those requirements and the Sentinel Initiative and the unique device identification (UDI) system, which are both under development, as well as CDRH compliance and enforcement actions.

## Labeling

Like drugs and biological products, all FDA approved or cleared medical devices are required to be labeled in a way that informs a user of how to use the device. The FFDCA defines a "label" as a "display of written, printed, or graphic matter upon the immediate container of any article."[73] "Labeling" is defined as "all labels and other written, printed, or graphic matter upon any article or any of its containers or wrappers, or accompanying such article" at any time while a device is held for sale after shipment or delivery for shipment in interstate commerce.[74]

---

[70] 21 CFR 14.

[71] FDA, *FY2010 Performance Report to the Congress for the Medical Device User Fee Amendments of 2007*, http://www.fda.gov/downloads/AboutFDA/ReportsManualsForms/Reports/UserFeeReports/PerformanceReports/MDUFMA/UCM243386.pdf. See also 21 CFR 814.40.

[72] FDA officials meet with industry leaders to agree upon mutually acceptable fee types, amounts, exceptions, and performance goals. The agreement specifies that, in return for the additional resources provided by medical device user fees, FDA is expected to meet performance goals defined in a letter, generally referred to as the "FDA Commitment Letter," from the HHS Secretary to the Chairmen and Ranking Minority Members of the Committee on Health, Education, Labor and Pensions of the U.S. Senate and the Committee on Energy and Commerce of the U.S. House of Representatives. This process is similar to the one used for prescription drug user fees under the Prescription Drug User Fee Act (PDUFA). For further information on PDUFA, see CRS Report RL33914, *The Prescription Drug User Fee Act History Through the 2007 PDUFA IV Reauthorization*, by Susan Thaul.

[73] FFDCA §201(k)

[74] FFDCA §201(m)

The term "accompanying" is interpreted to mean more than physical association with the product; it extends to posters, tags, pamphlets, circulars, booklets, brochures, instruction books, direction sheets, fillers, webpages, etc. Accompanying can also include labeling that is connected with the device after shipment or delivery for shipment in interstate commerce. According to an appellate court decision, "most, if not all advertising, is labeling. The term 'labeling' is defined in the FFDCA as including all printed matter accompanying any article. Congress did not, and we cannot, exclude from the definition printed matter which constitutes advertising."[75]

All devices must conform to the general labeling requirements.[76] Certain devices require specific labeling which may include not only package labeling, but informational literature, patient release forms, performance testing, and/or specific tolerances or prohibitions on certain ingredients.[77]

A section of the QSR also has an impact on various aspects of labeling.[78] The QSR regulation applies to the application of labeling to ensure legibility under normal conditions of use over the expected life of the device and also applies to inspection, handling, storage, and distribution of labeling. FDA considers a device to be adulterated if these requirements are not met. These requirements do not apply to the adequacy of labeling content, except to make sure the content meets labeling specifications contained in the device master record. However, failure to comply with GMP requirements, such as proofreading and change control, could result in labeling content errors. In such cases, the device could be misbranded and/or adulterated.

## Manufacturing

Like drug manufacturers, medical device manufacturers must produce their devices in accordance with Good Manufacturing Practice (GMP). The GMP requirements for devices are described in the QSR.[79] The QSRs require that domestic or foreign manufacturers have a quality system for the design, manufacture, packaging, labeling, storage, installation, and servicing of non-exempt finished medical devices intended for commercial distribution in the United States. The regulation requires that various specifications and controls be established for devices; that devices be designed and manufactured under a quality system to meet these specifications; that finished devices meet these specifications; that devices be correctly installed, checked and serviced; that quality data be analyzed to identify and correct quality problems; and that complaints be processed. FDA monitors device problem data and inspects the operations and records of device developers and manufacturers to determine compliance with the GMP requirements.[80] Though FDA has identified in QSR the essential elements that a quality system should have, manufacturers have a great deal of leeway to design quality systems that best cover nuances of their devices and the means of producing them.

---

[75] United States v. Research Laboratories, Inc., 126 F.2d 42 (9th Cir. 1942).

[76] 21 CFR 801

[77] 21 CFR 801.405 to 801.437. Denture repair kits, impact resistant lenses in sunglasses and eyeglasses, ozone emission levels, chlorofluorocarbon propellants, hearing aids, menstrual tampons, chlorofluorocarbons or other ozone depleting substances, latex condoms, and devices containing natural rubber.

[78] 21 CFR 820.120

[79] FFDCA §520; 21 CFR 820

[80] FDA, *Medical Devices 1. The Quality System Regulation*, June 18, 2009, http://www.fda.gov/MedicalDevices/ DeviceRegulationandGuidance/PostmarketRequirements/QualitySystemsRegulations/ MedicalDeviceQualitySystemsManual/ucm122391.htm.

## Postmarketing Surveillance

The 2011 IOM report states that because "it is not possible to create a premarket review process that could completely ensure the safety of all devices before they enter the market, a strong surveillance system that monitors the safety of medical devices is essential. The identification of problems associated with a medical device can be an opportunity for various corrective actions."[81] Such actions might include changing the device labeling and instructions for use, improving user training, or removal of the device from the market if appropriate. While the term postmarketing surveillance refers to a wide range of programs, the term postmarket surveillance refers to a specific activity defined in law.[82]

### Postmarket Surveillance

For certain devices introduced into interstate commerce after January 1, 1991, manufacturers must conduct postmarket surveillance studies, once their device is approved or cleared for marketing, in order to gather safety and efficacy data. This requirement applies to devices that

- are permanent implants, the failure of which may cause serious adverse health consequences or death;

- are intended for use in supporting or sustaining human life; or

- present a potential serious risk to human health.

FDA may require postmarket surveillance for other devices if deemed necessary to protect the public health. The primary objective of postmarket surveillance is to study the performance of the device after clearance or approval as it is used in the population for which it is intended—and to discover cases of device failure and its attendant impact on the patient. Manufacturers may receive notification that their device is subject to postmarket surveillance when FDA files (i.e., accepts) the submission, and again when a final decision is made. If notified, manufacturers must submit a plan for postmarket surveillance to FDA for approval within 30 days of introducing their device into interstate commerce. MDUFA authorized the appropriation of $25 million per year for Postmarket Studies and Surveillance.[83]

### Adverse Event Reporting

The Safe Medical Devices Act of 1990 (SMDA, P.L. 101-629) required FDA to establish a system for monitoring and tracking serious adverse events that resulted from the use or misuse of medical devices.[84] The Medical Device Reporting (MDR) regulation is the mechanism that FDA and manufacturers use to identify and monitor significant adverse events involving medical devices, so that problems are detected and corrected in a timely manner.[85]

---

[81] IOM, *Medical Devices and the Public's Health  The FDA 510(k) Clearance Process at 35 Years*, Washington, DC, July 2011, p. 99.

[82] FFDCA §522.

[83] 21 USC 355 note

[84] FFDCA §519(a)

[85] The searchable MDR database for devices is publically accessible at http://www.accessdata.fda.gov/scripts/cdrh/cfdocs/cfmdr/search.CFM.

Device manufacturers are required to report to FDA (1) within 30 calendar days of acquiring information that reasonably suggests one of their devices may have caused or contributed to a death, serious injury, or malfunction and (2) within 5 working days if an event requires action other than routine maintenance or service to prevent a public health issue.[86] User facilities, such as hospitals and nursing homes, are also required to report deaths to both the manufacturer, if known, and FDA within 10 working days.[87] User facilities must report serious injuries to the manufacturers (or FDA if the manufacturer is unknown) within 10 working days.[88] User facilities must also submit annual reports to FDA of all adverse event reports sent to manufacturers or FDA in the past year.[89]

In August 2009, FDA published notice of a proposed rule, and a related draft guidance document, that would require manufacturers to submit MDRs to the agency in an electronic format.[90] According to FDA, the proposed regulatory changes would provide the agency with a more efficient data entry process that would allow for timely access to medical device adverse event information and identification of emerging public health issues. The device industry requested a longer timeframe to implement the changes.

An October 2009 HHS Office of Inspector General report raised a number of questions about adverse event reporting for medical devices.[91] The report found that CDRH does not consistently use adverse event reporting and made several recommendations about how it could better do so.

## Medical Device Tracking

Manufacturers are required to track certain devices from their manufacture through the distribution chain when they receive an order from FDA to implement a tracking system for a certain type of device.[92] The purpose of device tracking is to ensure that manufacturers of these devices can locate them quickly once in commercial distribution if needed to facilitate notifications and recalls in the case of serious risks to health presented by the devices. FDA may issue a tracking order for any Class II or Class III device:

- the failure of which would be reasonably likely to have serious adverse health consequences;

- which is intended to be implanted in the human body for more than one year; or

---

[86] 21 CFR 803.10(c)(1) and 803.10(c)(2)

[87] 21 CFR 803.10(a)(1)(i).

[88] 21 CFR 803.10(a)(1)(ii).

[89] 21 CFR 803.10(a)(2) and 803.33.

[90] FDA, "Proposed Rule, Medical Device Reporting: Electronic Submission Requirements," 74 *Federal Register* 42203-42217, August 21, 2009; and FDA, "Draft Guidance for Industry, User Facilities, and Food and Drug Administration Staff; eMDR—Electronic Medical Device Reporting; Availability," 74 *Federal Register* Page 42310, August 21, 2009.

[91] Daniel R. Levinson, *Adverse Event Reporting for Medical Devices*, HHS Office of Inspector General, OEI-01-08-00110, October 2009, http://oig.hhs.gov/oei/reports/oei-01-08-00110.pdf.

[92] FDA, *Medical Device Tracking*, May 13, 2009, http://www.fda.gov/MedicalDevices/DeviceRegulationandGuidance/PostmarketRequirements/MedicalDeviceTracking/default.htm#link_2.

---

- which is intended to be a life sustaining or life supporting device used outside a device user facility.[93]

FDA has issued orders to track 13 implantable devices (including silicone gel-filled breast implants, various joint prostheses, implantable pacemakers, implantable defibrillator, mechanical heart valves, and implantable infusion pumps) and four other devices that are used outside a device user facility.[94]

## The Sentinel Initiative

Section 905 of FDAAA mandated that FDA create an active postmarket risk identification system.[95] Although the FDAAA language is focused on monitoring drugs, FDA is using its general authority to monitor all FDA-regulated products, including medical devices, after they have reached the market.[96] FDA launched the Sentinel Initiative in May 2008; once completed, it will be called the Sentinel System. FDAAA set goals that the new system must be able to access data on 25 million people by July 2010, a goal which FDA has met, and 100 million people by July 2012.[97] As of January 2011 FDA has the capacity to access data from the electronic health records of more than 60 million people.[98]

FDA is collaborating with institutions throughout the United States, including academic medical centers, healthcare systems and health insurance companies, who act as data partners in the system. Additional collaborators will include patient and healthcare professional advocacy groups, academic institutions and the medical products industry. As an example of data applicable to medical devices, "one Sentinel-related project identified, described, and evaluated potential US orthopedic-implant registries that could participate in the creation of a national network of such registries as part of the Sentinel Initiative. Data related to medical devices include rates of selected outcomes (for example, myocardial infarction and stroke), rates of infection, and rates of implant revision and reintervention."[99] According to FDA, the Sentinel Initiative aims to develop and implement a proactive system that will complement existing systems that the agency has in place to track reports of adverse events linked to the use of its regulated products.[100]

---

[93] 21 CFR 821

[94] A device user facility means a hospital, ambulatory surgical facility, nursing home, or outpatient treatment facility which is not a physician's office. A current list of the devices for which tracking is required can be found at http://www.fda.gov/MedicalDevices/DeviceRegulationandGuidance/PostmarketRequirements/MedicalDeviceTracking/default.htm#link_2.

[95] FFDCA §505(k); 21 USC 355

[96] FFDCA §1003(b)(2)(c)

[97] U.S. Food and Drug Administration, *The Sentinel Initiative Access to Electronic Healthcare Data for More Than 25 Million Lives*, July 2010, http://www.fda.gov/downloads/Safety/FDAsSentinelInitiative/UCM233360.pdf.

[98] Rachel E. Behrman, Joshua S. Benner, and Jeffrey S. Brown, et al., "Developing the Sentinel System—A National Resource for Evidence Development," *The New England Journal of Medicine*, vol. 364, no. 6 (February 10, 2011), pp. 498-499. The Sentinel Initiative is focused on electronic claims data held by health plans. Importantly, the plans retain control over the patient-level data within their own data firewalls and provide only aggregated information to FDA.

[99] IOM, *Medical Devices and the Public's Health The FDA 510(k) Clearance Process at 35 Years*, Washington, DC, July 2011, p. 106.

[100] Information on the current status of the Sentinel Initiative is available at http://www.fda.gov/Safety/FDAsSentinelInitiative/default.htm.

---

## Unique Device Identification

A provision in FDAAA requires the HHS Secretary to promulgate regulations establishing a unique device identification (UDI) system.[101] When implemented, this new system will require

- the label of a device to bear a unique identifier, unless an alternative location is specified by FDA or unless an exception is made for a particular device or group of devices;

- the unique identifier to be able to identify the device through distribution and use; and

- the unique identifier to include the lot or serial number if specified by FDA.

According to FDA, "incorporation of UDI into various health-related databases will greatly facilitate many important public health-related activities including: reducing medical errors; reporting and assessing device-related adverse events and product problems; tracking of recalls; assessing patient-centered outcomes and the risk/benefit profile of medical devices in large segments of the U.S. population; and, providing an easily accessible source of device identification information to patients and health care professionals."[102]

CDRH indicated in its FY2010 Strategic Priorities that the UDI system will be implemented by September 30, 2013.[103] UDI will be implemented in three phases: Class III devices will need to be in compliance within one year after the final rule is published, Class II at three years and Class I at five years after the final rule.[104] FDA has held a number of public meetings and workshops with stakeholders to discuss the adoption, implementation, and use of a UDI system. The agency has posted on its website information about these meetings as well as a number of reports on the use of UDI for medical devices.[105]

FDA has been working with the Global Harmonization Task Force (GHTF) to foster international harmonization in the regulation of medical devices through the development of non-binding guidance documents.[106] The GHTF is a voluntary international group of representatives from medical device regulatory authorities and trade associations from Europe, the United States, Canada, Japan and Australia. In September 2011 the GHTF published its final document on UDI for medical devices.[107]

---

[101] FFDCA §519(f); 21 USC 360i

[102] FDA, "Unique Device Identification for Postmarket Surveillance and Enforcement; Public Workshop," 76 *Federal Register* 43691-43693, July 21, 2011.

[103] FDA, Center for Devices and Radiological Health, *CDRH FY 2010 Strategic Priorities*, p. 6, http://www.fda.gov/downloads/AboutFDA/CentersOffices/CDRH/CDRHVisionandMission/UCM197648.pdf.

[104] Alaina Bush, "CER, Safety uses eyed as part of FDA device identification rule," *Inside Health Reform*, vol. 3, no. 39 (September 22, 2011).

[105] Meeting information, reports and current status of the UDI system can be found at http://www.fda.gov/MedicalDevices/DeviceRegulationandGuidance/UniqueDeviceIdentification/default.htm

[106] GHTF website is at http://www.ghtf.org/.

[107] GHTF SC UDI Ad Hoc Working Group, *Unique Device Identification (UDI) System for Medical Devices*, Global Harmonization Task Force, GHTF/AHWG-UDI/N2R3:2011, September 16, 2011, http://www.ghtf.org/documents/ahwg/AHWG-UDI-N2R3.pdf.

## Compliance and Enforcement

Compliance requirements apply to both the premarket approval process and postmarket surveillance. When a problem arises with a product regulated by FDA, the agency can take a number of actions to protect the public health. Initially, the agency tries to work with the manufacturer to correct the problem on a voluntary basis. If that fails, legal remedies may be taken, such as: asking the manufacturer to recall a product, having federal marshals seize products, or detaining imports at the port of entry until problems are corrected. If warranted, FDA can ask the courts to issue injunctions or prosecute individual company officers that deliberately violate the law. When warranted, criminal penalties, including prison sentences, may be sought.

Section 516 of the FFDCA gives FDA the authority to ban devices that present substantial deception or unreasonable and substantial risk of illness or injury. Section 518 enables FDA to require manufacturers or other appropriate individuals to notify all health professionals who prescribe or use the device and any other person (including manufacturers, importers, distributors, retailers, and device users) of any health risks resulting from the use of a violative device, so that these risks may be reduced or eliminated. This section also gives consumers a procedure for economic redress when they have been sold defective medical devices that present unreasonable risks. Section 519 of the act authorized FDA to promulgate regulations requiring manufacturers, importers, and distributors of devices to maintain records and reports to assure that devices are not adulterated or misbranded. Section 520(e) authorizes FDA to restrict the sale, distribution, or use of a device if there cannot otherwise be reasonable assurance of its safety and effectiveness. A restricted device can only be sold on oral or written authorization by a licensed practitioner or under conditions specified by regulation.

### Inspection

Each FDA center has an Office of Compliance (OC) that ensures compliance with regulations while pre- or postmarket studies are being undertaken, with manufacturing requirements, and with labeling requirements. The objectives of CDRH's OC's Bioresearch Monitoring (BIMO) program are to ensure the quality and integrity of data and information submitted in support of IDE, PMA, and 510(k) submissions and to ensure that human subjects taking part in investigations are protected from undue hazard or risk. This is achieved through audits of clinical data contained in PMAs prior to approval, data audits of IDE and 510(k) submissions, inspections of IRBs and nonclinical laboratories, and enforcement of the prohibitions against promotion, marketing, or commercialization of investigational devices. Any establishment where devices are manufactured, processed, packed, installed, used, or implanted or where records of results from use of devices are kept, can be subject to inspection. (See **Table 2**.)

**Table 2. CDRH, FDA Foreign and Domestic Inspections, FY2004–FY2010**

| | FY | 2004 | 2005 | 2006 | 2007 | 2008 | 2009 | 2010 |
|---|---|---|---|---|---|---|---|---|
| **Number of Inspections** | | 2,936 | 2,694 | 2,691 | 2,495 | 2,353 | 2,550 | 3,174 |

**Source:** FDA Center for Devices and Radiological Health, Office of Compliance, Division of Risk Management Operations based on Center Ad Hoc Reporting System inspection data.

The OC also reviews the quality system design and manufacturing information in the PMA submission to determine whether the manufacturer has described the processes in sufficient detail and to make a preliminary determination of whether the manufacturer meets the QSR. If the manufacturer has provided an adequate description of the design and manufacturing process, a preapproval inspection can be initiated. Inspection is to include an assessment of the manufacturer's capability to design and manufacture the device as claimed in the PMA and confirm that the quality system is in compliance with the QSR. Postapproval inspections can be conducted within 8 to 12 months of approval of the PMA submission. The inspection is to primarily focus on any changes that may have been made in the device design, manufacturing process, or quality systems.

The compliance offices work closely with the Office of Regulatory Affairs (ORA),[108] which operates in the field to regulate almost 124,000 business establishments that annually produce, warehouse, import and transport $1 trillion worth of medical products. Consumer safety officers (CSOs) and inspectors typically have conducted about 22,000 domestic and foreign inspections a year to ensure that regulated products meet the agency's standards. CSOs also monitor clinical trials. Scientists in ORA's 13 laboratories typically have analyzed more than 41,000 product samples each year to determine their adherence to FDA's standards.

## Warning Letter

A warning letter is a written communication from FDA notifying a responsible individual, manufacturer, or facility that the agency considers one or more products, practices, processes, or other activities to be in violation of the laws that FDA enforces. The warning letter informs the recipient that failure to take appropriate and prompt action to correct and prevent any future repeat of the violations could result in an administrative or regulatory action. Although serious noncompliance is often a catalyst for issuance of a warning letter, the warning letter is informal and advisory.[109] (See **Table 3**.)

**Table 3. CDRH Warning Letters Issued, FY2000–FY2010**

| FY | 2000 | 2001 | 2002 | 2003 | 2004 | 2005 | 2006 | 2007 | 2008 | 2009 | 2010 |
|---|---|---|---|---|---|---|---|---|---|---|---|
| **Number of Letters** | 528 | 498 | 285 | 205 | 198 | 182 | 154 | 155 | 152 | 136 | 204 |

**Source:** FDA Center for Devices and Radiological Health, Office of Compliance, Division of Risk Management Operations based on Office of Regulatory Affairs Case Management System warning letter data.

## Product Recall

A recall is a method of removing or correcting products that FDA considers are in violation of the law.[110] Medical device recalls are usually conducted voluntarily by the manufacturer after

---

[108] See ORA at http://www.fda.gov/AboutFDA/CentersOffices/ORA/default.htm.

[109] Warning letters are publically available on FDA's website at http://www.fda.gov/ICECI/EnforcementActions/ WarningLetters/default.htm.

[110] Recall does not include market withdrawal or a stock recovery. A market withdrawal is a firm's removal or correction of a distributed product for a minor violation that does not violate the law and would not be subject to legal action by FDA (e.g., normal stock rotation practices, routine equipment adjustments and repairs, etc.). Stock recovery involves correction of a problem before product is shipped (i.e., is still in the manufacturer's control).

negotiation with FDA.[111] Manufacturers (including refurbishers and reconditioners) and importers are required to report to FDA any correction or removal of a medical device that is undertaken to reduce a health risk posed by the device.[112] A recall may be a total market withdrawal or may be of a portion of product (such as a single lot). In rare instances, where the manufacturer or importer fails to voluntarily recall a device that is a risk to health, FDA may issue a recall order to the manufacturer.[113]

When a recall is initiated, FDA performs an evaluation of the health hazard presented taking into account the following factors, among others:

- Whether any disease or injuries have occurred from the use of the product;

- Whether any existing conditions could contribute to a clinical situation that could expose humans or animals to a health hazard;

- Assessment of hazard to various populations (e.g., children, surgical patients, pets, livestock) who would be exposed to the product;

- Assessment of the degree of seriousness of the health hazard to which the populations at risk would be exposed;

- Assessment of the likelihood of occurrence of the hazard;

- Assessment of the consequences (immediate or long-range) of the hazard.

Following the health hazard assessment, FDA assigns the recall a classification according to the relative degree of health hazard. *Class I* recalls are the most serious, reserved for situations where there is a reasonable probability that the use of, or exposure to, a product will cause serious adverse health consequences or death. *Class II* recalls are for situations where the use of, or exposure to, a product may cause temporary or medically reversible adverse health consequences or where the probability of serious adverse health consequences is remote. In a *Class III* recall situation, the use of, or exposure to, a product is not likely to cause adverse health consequences. (See **Table 4**.) In addition to a warning letter or recall, FDA may issue a public notification or safety alert (e.g., "Dear Doctor" letter), to warn healthcare providers and consumers of the risk of the device.[114]

**Table 4. CDRH Class I, II, and III Product Recalls, FY2004–FY2010**

| FY | 2004 | 2005 | 2006 | 2007 | 2008 | 2009 | 2010 |
|---|---|---|---|---|---|---|---|
| Class I | 36 | 77 | 76 | 45 | 131 | 219 | 334 |
| Class II | 1,235 | 1,351 | 1,252 | 1,102 | 2,178 | 2,222 | 2,208 |
| Class III | 219 | 170 | 222 | 132 | 163 | 194 | 92 |

**Source:** FDA Center for Devices and Radiological Health, Office of Compliance, Division of Risk Management Operations based on Center Ad Hoc Reporting System recall data.

---

[111] 21 CFR 7

[112] 21 CFR 806.

[113] 21 CFR 810. See out-of-print CRS Report RL34167, *The FDA's Authority to Recall Products*, by Vanessa K. Burrows (available from the author upon request).

[114] The main page for recalls, market withdrawals, and safety alerts for all FDA-regulated products is http://www.fda.gov/opacom/7alerts.html.

# Appendix A. History of Laws Governing Medical Device Regulation

## The Federal Food, Drug and Cosmetics Act of 1938

The first general federal food and drug law, the *Food and Drugs Act of 1906*, did not contain any provisions to regulate medical device safety or claims made regarding such devices. Strong support for reform developed during the 1930s due to "false therapeutic claims for medical devices [that] were being presented to the public through radio and newspaper advertising."[115] Medical devices came under federal scrutiny when Congress passed the *Federal Food, Drug and Cosmetic Act (FFDCA) of 1938* (P.L. 75-717). The regulatory authority provided to FDA by the 1938 law was "limited to action after a medical device has been offered for introduction into interstate commerce" and only when the device was deemed to be "adulterated or misbranded."[116]

Most of the legitimate devices on the market at the time the 1938 Act became law "were relatively simple items which applied basic science concepts such that experts using them could readily recognize whether the device was functioning properly; the major concern with respect to these devices was assuring truthful labeling."[117] During the first 20 years following enactment of the 1938 law, FDA's activity with respect to medical devices involved protecting the American public from *fraudulent* devices; FDA began to turn its attention to the hazards from *legitimate* devices around 1960.[118]

> The post-war revolution in biomedical technology had resulted in the introduction of a wide variety of sophisticated devices. New developments in the electronic, plastic, metallurgy, and ceramics industries, coupled with progress in design engineering, led to invention of the heart pacemaker, the kidney dialysis machine, defibrillators, cardiac and renal catheters, surgical implants, artificial vessels and heart valves, intensive care monitoring units, and a wide spectrum of other diagnostic and therapeutic devices. Although many lives have been saved or improved by the new discoveries, the potential for harm to consumers has been heightened by the critical medical conditions in which sophisticated modern devices are used and by the complicated technology involved in their manufacture and use. In the search to expand medical knowledge, new experimental approaches have sometimes been tried without adequate premarket clinical testing, quality control in materials selected, or patient consent.[119]

The Dalkon Shield, a contraceptive device introduced in November 1970, is "an example of a legitimate device which was marketed without adequate premarket testing."[120] Other examples

---

[115] U.S. Congress, House Committee on Interstate and Foreign Commerce, *Medical Device Amendments of 1976*, to accompany H.R. 11124, 94th Cong., 2nd sess., February 29, 1976, H. Rept. 94-853, p. 6.

[116] Ibid. "A device is adulterated if it includes any filthy, putrid, or decomposed substance, or if it is prepared, packed, or held under unsanitary conditions. A device is misbranded if its labeling is false or misleading; unless it identifies the manufacturer, packer, or distributor and quantity of contents; if required labeling statements are not conspicuous; if it fails to bear adequate directions for use or adequate warnings; or if it is dangerous to health when used as indicated."

[117] Ibid.

[118] Ibid., p. 7.

[119] Ibid., p. 7-8.

[120] Ibid., p. 8. By 1975, the Dalkon Shield had been linked to at least 16 deaths and 25 miscarriages, numerous cases of (continued...)

---

include defective cardiac pacemakers and intraocular lenses which, following implantation, caused unusual eye infections resulting in serious vision impairment or the need for removal of the eye.

Congress amended the FFDCA in 1962 to require FDA approval of a new drug application prior to marketing and to require that a new drug be shown to be effective as well as safe. Following these changes, FDA began "to impose rigorous premarket approval of some products that today would be deemed devices." Court decisions in the late 1960s upheld FDA's authority to regulate some medical devices as drugs due in part to the overlapping definitions of drug and device in the 1938 law. FDA classified a number of devices as drugs (contact lenses, injectable silicone, pregnancy-test kits, bone cement), and only such devices were subject to premarket review (prior to 1976). However the approach of classifying devices as a drug was unsuccessful in other court decisions and the need for more comprehensive authority to regulate devices was recognized by the Kennedy, Johnson and Nixon administrations.[121]

## The Medical Device Amendments of 1976

The *Medical Device Amendments of 1976* (MDA; P.L. 94-295) was the first major legislation passed to address the review of medical devices. The MDA provided a definition for the term device.[122] It established a number of requirements referred to as *general controls* that applied to all devices.[123] Examples include provisions on adulteration and misbranding, prohibitions on false or misleading advertising, and a requirement to register all medical device manufacturers with FDA. One such provision required manufacturers to notify FDA 90 days prior to the marketing of any new device; if the agency failed to act, marketing could begin. Because this provision is outlined in section 510(k) of the FFDCA, it is often referred to as a "510(k) notification."

The MDA directed FDA to classify, into one of three classes, all medical devices that were on the market at the time of enactment; these are the *preamendment* devices.[124] Congress provided

---

(...continued)

pelvic perforation and pelvic infection, removal of the IUD for medical reasons, and pregnancies due to IUD failure. As of February 1976, more than 500 lawsuits seeking compensatory and punitive damages totaling more than $400 million were pending against the manufacturer of the Dalkon Shield. IOM, *Medical Devices and the Public's Health The FDA 510(k) Clearance Process at 35 Years*, Washington, DC, July 2011, p. 172, http://www.iom.edu/Reports/2011/Medical-Devices-and-the-Publics-Health-The-FDA-510k-Clearance-Process-at-35-Years.aspx.

[121] U.S. Congress, House Committee on Interstate and Foreign Commerce, *Medical Device Amendments of 1976*, to accompany H.R. 11124, 94th Cong., 2nd sess., February 29, 1976, H. Rept. 94-853, p. 8-9.

[122] An instrument, apparatus, implement, machine, contrivance, implant, in vitro reagent, or other similar or related article, including any component, part, or accessory, which is (1) recognized in the official National Formulary, or the United States Pharmacopeia, or any supplement to them; (2) intended for use in the diagnosis of disease or other conditions, or in the cure, mitigation, treatment, or prevention of disease, in man or other animals; or (3) intended to affect the structure or any function of the body of man or other animals, and which does not achieve any of its principal intended purposes through chemical action within or on the body of man or other animals and which is not dependent upon being metabolized for the achievement of its primary intended purposes. The definition was changed in 1992 from "any of its principal intended purposes" to "its primary intended purposes." Current definition at FFDCA §201(h), (21 U.S.C. 321).

[123] The law has since been amended to exempt many (Class I) products from some general controls or to limit the application of general controls to subsets of (Class II or Class III) products that pose higher risks. IOM, *Medical Devices and the Public's Health The FDA 510(k) Clearance Process at 35 Years*, Washington, DC, July 2011, p. 175.

[124] Preamendment devices were presumed to be marketable. They did not undergo premarket review and could be legally marketed unless FDA required their removal. After classifying the preamendment devices, FDA used them as (continued...)

---

definitions for the three classes—Class I, Class II, Class III—based on the risks to patients posed by the devices. In contrast to the approach taken with pharmaceuticals (all, except generic agents, undergo rigorous premarket review and approval), Congress limited premarket approval to only a small number of devices. "Only the highest-risk category [Class III] would require agency review and approval as a precondition for commercial sale and routine medical use. The other two categories would be subject not to a rigorous review but merely a requirement [510(k)] that the manufacturer of a device notify FDA, at least 90 days before commencing marketing, of its intent to distribute the product commercially."[125] For Class I devices, no additional review was needed once the status of Class I was confirmed; general controls were considered to be sufficient to protect public health. For Class II devices, limited supplemental review would be needed to verify conformity with performance standards if such standards had been established by the agency.[126]

Under MDA, all devices coming to market after enactment were automatically placed in Class III until reclassified; these are the *postamendment* devices. As stated above, Class III medical devices receive more intense scrutiny and require an application for premarket approval (PMA) before the device can be marketed. However, the MDA allowed for the reclassification of a device from one class to another. According to a 2011 IOM report on medical devices:

> The classification and reclassification process did not include any evaluation of the safety or effectiveness of the device types being categorized. Once a device type was assigned to Class III, the FDA was directed to promulgate a regulation calling for manufacturers of devices of that type to submit a [PMA] application. The agency would then (and only then) undertake a review of the safety and effectiveness of the devices. For device types placed into Class I or Class II, there was no mechanism for the systematic review of safety and effectiveness. Congress envisioned instead that the agency would use its postmarketing tools to identify and address issues of lack of safety or lack of effectiveness case by case. Thus, preamendment devices in Class I and II were never subjected to a comprehensive FDA evaluation for safety or effectiveness. The classification process was not completed until 1988.[127]

For postamendment devices, which were automatically placed into Class III, there were two important exceptions:

> The primary exception involved a postamendment device that was substantially equivalent to another device of the same type that either as a preamendment device that had not been classified into any class or was not a preamendment device but had already been classified into Class I or Class II. The FDA permitted manufacturers of postamendment devices to demonstrate substantial equivalence to a preamendment device in Class I or II as part of the 510(k) submission. An alternative exception provided that the postamendment device would not be in Class III if the FDA, in response to a petition, classified it into Class I or Class II.[128]

The MDA did not provide a definition for the term *substantially equivalent.* The MDA also did not itemize the required contents of a 510(k). Such a notification "need only set forth its proposed

---

(...continued)

the first cadre of "predicate" devices in order to demonstrate substantial equivalence.

[125] Ibid., p. 24.

[126] Ibid., p. 177.

[127] Ibid., p. 25.

[128] Ibid., p. 179.

intended use or indications for use, the device to which substantial equivalence is claimed, and evidence demonstrating that equivalence."[129]

## The Safe Medical Devices Act of 1990

The *Safe Medical Devices Act of 1990* (SMDA; P.L. 101-629) made a number of changes to the law such as providing a definition for the term *substantial equivalence* and revising the definition for Class II. FDA had not promulgated performance standards for most Class II devices. The new law authorized the use of alternative restrictions, called special controls, at the agency's discretion and simplified the process of establishing performance standards for Class II devices. Examples of special controls include special labeling requirements, mandatory performance standards, patient registries and postmarket surveillance.

FDA also had experienced difficulty in promulgating regulations needed to require submission of PMA applications for Class III devices. SMDA authorized FDA to reconsider all the preamendment devices that had been placed in Class III and reclassify some of these devices into Class I or Class II.[130] The purpose was "to reduce the number of device types that needed PMA review."[131] For those devices remaining in Class III, the agency was directed to establish a schedule for promulgation of regulations calling for PMAs of devices that still used the 510(k) notification as an entry to the marketplace.

Under SMDA, FDA must issue a response to a 510(k) submission before marketing of a new device can begin. SMDA allowed for the evaluation of safety and effectiveness data in 510(k) notifications, but only in certain situations. These were limited to cases in which a new device offered different technologic characteristics from the already marketed *premendment or postamendment* (predicate) device.[132] "Because the assessment of substantial equivalence generally did not

> **U.S. Supreme Court 1996 Opinion Medtronic v. Lohr**
>
> "Substantial equivalence determinations provide little protection to the public. These determinations simply compare a post-1976 device to a pre-1976 device to ascertain whether the latter is no more dangerous and no less effective than the earlier device. If the earlier device poses a severe risk or is ineffective, then the latter device may also be risky or ineffective."
> Medtronic, Inc. v. Lohr, 518 U.S. 470 (1996).

require evidence of safety or effectiveness of a device and because a preamendment device to which equivalence was established was not itself reviewed for safety or effectiveness, the FDA made clear from the outset that clearance of a 510(k) notification was not a determination that the cleared device was safe or effective. That position was reiterated by the agency numerous times. The US Supreme Court accepted this interpretation in a 1996 opinion."[133]

SMDA established postmarket requirements for medical devices. SMDA required facilities that use medical devices to report to FDA any incident that suggested that a medical device could

---

[129] Ibid. p. 180.

[130] FFDCA §515(i).

[131] IOM, *Medical Devices and the Public's Health The FDA 510(k) Clearance Process at 35 Years*, Washington, DC, July 2011, p. 205.

[132] FFDCA §513(i).

[133] IOM, *Medical Devices and the Public's Health The FDA 510(k) Clearance Process at 35 Years*, Washington, DC, July 2011, p. 28.

have caused or contributed to the death, serious illness, or injury of a patient. Manufacturers of certain permanently implanted devices were required to establish methods for tracking the patients who received them and to conduct postmarket surveillance to identify adverse events. The act authorized FDA to carry out certain enforcement actions, such as device product recalls, for products that did not comply with the law.

## The Food and Drug Administration Modernization Act of 1997

The *Food and Drug Administration Modernization Act of 1997* (FDAMA; P.L. 105-115) mandated wide-ranging reforms in the regulation of foods, drugs and medical devices by FDA. In general, provisions involving medical devices "were designed to reduce FDA's workload and permit concentration of resources on devices that presented greater potential for harm" and "to limit the FDA's discretion and authority in regulating the device industry" in order to "accelerate the pace of technology transfer."[134]

FDAMA eliminated the 510(k) notification requirement for most Class I devices and some Class II devices. It authorized the creation of a third-party review system of 510(k) submissions for Class I and most Class II devices that still required 510(k) review. It allowed certain new devices (those not substantially equivalent to another device and automatically placed in Class III) to be evaluated for immediate placement in Class I or Class II. This process, called the de novo 510(k), avoids PMA review, must be completed in 60 days, and may be requested by the sponsor.

For substantial equivalence determinations in which the new device has a different technological characteristic, FDAMA requires that FDA "consider the least burdensome means of demonstrating substantial equivalence and request information accordingly."[135] For a medical device using an important breakthrough technology, or which does not have an approved alternative device, priority review of the PMA must be provided by FDA.[136]

FDAMA limited the use of some postmarket controls (device tracking and postmarket surveillance) to Class II and Class III devices, eased reporting requirements of adverse events for device user facilities, eliminated mandatory reporting of adverse events by medical device distributors, and directed FDA to establish a sentinel reporting system to collect information on deaths and serious injuries or illnesses associated with the use of a medical device.[137]

## User Fee Acts and the FDA Amendments Act of 2007

The *Medical Device User Fee and Modernization Act of 2002* (MDUFMA; P.L. 107-250) established a user fee program for premarket reviews of 510(k) submissions and PMA applications; user fees may not be used for other FDA or CDRH activities. MDUFMA also made targeted changes that would reduce regulatory burdens and agency workload, such as allowing establishment inspections to be conducted by accredited persons (third parties). MDUFMA was amended and clarified by two laws: the *Medical Device Technical Corrections Act of 2004*

---

[134] Ibid., p. 213.

[135] FFDCA §513(i)(1)(D).

[136] FFDCA §515(d)(5).

[137] FFDCA §519 and §522. A device user facility means a hospital, ambulatory surgical facility, nursing home, or outpatient treatment facility which is not a physician's office.

(MDTCA, P.L. 108-214), and the *Medical Device User Fee Stabilization Act of 2005* (MDUFSA, P.L. 109-43), and had its user fee provisions reauthorized by the *Medical Device User Fee Act of 2007* (MDUFA; Title II of FDAAA, see below).

The *Food and Drug Administration Amendments Act of 2007* (FDAAA; P.L. 110-85) amended the FFDCA and the Public Health Service Act to reauthorize several expiring programs (including the medical device user fee act) and to make agency-wide changes, several of which have implications for the regulation of medical devices.[138] FDAAA created incentives as well as reporting and safety requirements for manufacturers of medical devices for children; required that certain clinical trials for medical devices and some other products be publicly registered and have their results posted;[139] created requirements to reduce conflicts of interest in advisory committees for medical devices and other products;[140] and made certain other amendments to the regulation of devices.

---

[138] See CRS Report RL34465, *FDA Amendments Act of 2007 (P.L. 110-85)*, by Erin D. Williams and Susan Thaul.

[139] See the Clinical Trials Databases section of CRS Report RL34465, *FDA Amendments Act of 2007 (P.L. 110-85)*, by Erin D. Williams and Susan Thaul.

[140] FDA uses advisory committees to gain independent advice from outside experts. See CRS Report RS22691, *FDA Advisory Committee Conflict of Interest*, by Erin D. Williams.

# Appendix B. Acronyms Used in this Report

| | |
|---|---|
| **BIMO** | Bioresearch Monitoring |
| **CBER** | Center for Biologics Evaluation and Research |
| **CDRH** | Center for Devices and Radiological Health |
| **CFR** | Code of Federal Regulations |
| **CSOs** | Consumer safety officers |
| **FDA** | Food and Drug Administration |
| **FDAAA** | Food and Drug Administration Amendments Act of 2007 |
| **FDAMA** | Food and Drug Administration Modernization Act of 1997 |
| **FFDCA** | Federal Food, Drug and Cosmetic Act |
| **GAO** | General Accountability Office |
| **GGP** | Good Guidance Practices |
| **GHTF** | Global Harmonization Task Force |
| **GMP** | Good manufacturing practices |
| **HHS** | Health and Human Services |
| **IDE** | Investigational Device Exemption |
| **IOM** | Institute of Medicine |
| **IRB** | Institutional review board |
| **IVD** | In Vitro Diagnostic |
| **MDA** | Medical Device Amendments of 1976 |
| **MDR** | Medical Device Reporting |
| **MDTCA** | Medical Device Technical Corrections Act of 2004 |
| **MDUFA** | Medical Device User Fee Act of 2007 |
| **MDUFMA** | Medical Device User Fee and Modernization Act of 2002 |
| **MDUFSA** | Medical Device User Fee Stabilization Act of 2005 |
| **NSE** | Not substantially equivalent |
| **OC** | Office of Compliance |
| **ORA** | Office of Regulatory Affairs |
| **PMA** | Premarket Approval |
| **QSR** | Quality Systems Regulation |
| **SMDA** | Safe Medical Devices Act of 1990 |
| **UDI** | Unique device identification |

# Author Contact Information

Judith A. Johnson
Specialist in Biomedical Policy
jajohnson@crs.loc.gov, 7-7077